What they are saying about

Healing Journeys
Stories of Mind, Body & Spirit

"A heartfelt mixture of the physical and the metaphysical, the transformative and the healthful, from Chiropractic to the healing power of the body, mind and soul."

Dr John Demartini
Author of Count Your Blessings –
The Healing Power of Gratitude and Love

In this book, we learn that the physical symptom is usually just that...a symptom. The root cause is practically always emotional and must be discovered, acknowledged and dealt with in order for one to heal themselves. The wisdom of Dr. Kita can help us do just that and, as a result, live a happier, healthier, and more fulfilling life.

-Bob Burg
coauthor of The Go-Giver

A seemingly simple book with much wisdom, information, and a bit of magic. The book's central statement that "negative emotions can cause health problems" is not an unusual idea in itself, but Dr. Kevin Kita's handling is not just unusual but unique. ...Dr. Kita makes it fascinating by his plain and intelligent style. The author's unassuming and honest approach to each case and his deepening abilities inspire us. And, perhaps to our surprise

and, with that bit of magic, our authentic encounter with the author gives us an unexpected healing.

Lisa Nicole Woodside, PhD
Professor Emerita
Holy Family University

"This book is much like it's author – kind, gentle, thoughtful, helpful. ...Dr. Kita's work and book are truly holistic. It is fascinating to read about the interplay of body, thought, emotion, life-problems, and healing, in such simple, clear, compassionate writing. Nietzsche himself called attention to the powerful role of resentment in the modern psyche. (He also suffered from migraines and other debilitating problems which a gifted healer like Dr. Kita might have assuaged!)

Harold Weiss, Ph.D.
Professor of Philosophy
Northampton Community College

In this book, Dr. Kita demonstrates that a psychosomatic relationship does exist in the healing process. By compassionately listening to his patients he allows for a productive dialogue to ensue which brings to bear a mental or spiritual dimension to chiropractic care. The results may more readily affect a physical cure. In addition, this unique approach can only bring hope and encouragement to his patients. It's a great read!!!

Edward M. Murawski
Lecturer of Philosophy
La Salle University

Healing Journeys

Stories
of Mind, Body & Spirit

by

Dr. Kevin Kita

Illustrations
by
Jessie Krause

Healing Journeys
Stories of Mind, Body & Spirit

Copyright © 2014 by Dr. Kevin Kita.
ISBN: 978-0-9908210-0-7

The material in this book is not intended as a substitute for advice from physicians, therapists or other professionals. The reader should regularly consult his or her own physician in matters relating to health, exercise, diet or emotional well-being.

Names and identifying details of the patients, their family members and friends have been changed to protect the privacy of individuals.

Published by
Way of Life Press

Dedication

To all the patients and teachers who
have graciously allowed
me to learn from them.

Best wishes on your
Healing Journey.

K. Kitu

Acknowledgements

My deepest thanks go to my family for their unconditional love and acceptance for all that I do. Also, thanks to my extended family, Kristin Williams and Barbara Rose, for the insights that they shared with me, and to Jessie Krause who made the book beautiful.

Table of Contents

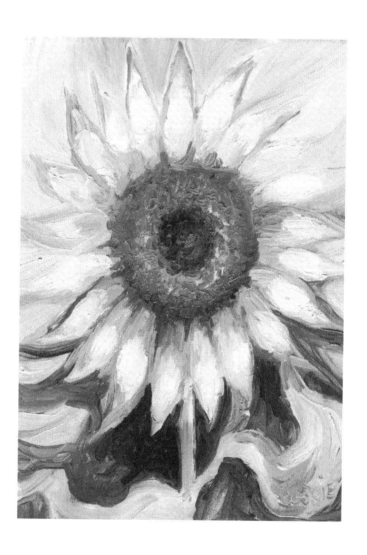

Introduction

I wrote this book at the urging of many of the patients who have come to my office seeking help. As I got to know them, and they me, they would tell me that I should write a book to share my experiences with people who are not able to visit me personally. I listened to their advice, and often thought about writing a book, but it took me years to finally sit down and begin to work on it.

Many people suffer from health problems that are caused by past emotional traumas or thinking patterns, but they have no understanding of the real, underlying cause of their physical symptoms, and so no way to really begin to heal. I hope that this book will help people to understand some of the things that I have learned in my own healing journey about the need to heal our emotional wounds in order to heal our physical symptoms.

My healing journey began by accident. I was still in Chiropractic College and during the small amount of spare time that I had, I would play tennis. I had played a lot of serious tennis in my youth and always considered myself to be in good physical shape. Then, at a weekend tennis tournament, I tore my right calf muscle. This puzzled me because I had never had any muscle issues in 25 years as a tennis player, or in any of the other sports I had participated in. I finished playing the match, and won it, even though I was in excruciating pain. I was supposed to play another match that day, but told the tournament director I couldn't play anymore.

After forfeiting the next match, I turned my attention to my calf muscle. It hurt a lot, but I wasn't worried because I had always healed fast. Little did I know that this time something would be different. I did the normal things one does for this type of injury, such as applying ice and resting it. One week went by and there was very little improvement. I was a bit surprised by this lack of improvement, but as things developed, this was only the beginning of my journey. Two weeks went by and no improvement. Three weeks passed and still no improvement. After a month my leg began to feel better, and I thought I was finally healed. I started to run on it, but I could only run one block before my calf muscle seized up again.

I was frustrated of course, and one day I mentioned my problem and my annoyance and frustration about it to one of my classmates. She suggested that I read a book by the well-known author and healer Louise Hay, titled *Heal Your Body*.

I read the book and learned the connection between our emotions and our body. Reading the book helped me to realize that I was in a state of fear about moving forward in my life: I was finishing Chiropractic College and I was terrified about opening my own practice. This fear was what was causing my calf muscle not to heal. As I realized the connection and dealt with my fear, my calf muscle finally began to heal quickly.

The healing journey I experienced at the start of my Chiropractic career taught me lessons that have helped me ever since in working with patients who have seemingly incurable ailments. It helped me to learn that often "incurable" really means that something must be cured from within ourselves.

Healing Journeys: Stories of Mind, Body & Spirit is comprised of just a few of the journeys that have begun in my office over the years. Some are hard to believe, even by me, but all of the events that I describe in this book have really happened. While they seem very surreal to me, they have also opened my eyes, and the eyes of the patients and their families and friends, to the power that our emotions have on our health.

As I experienced my own healing journey, and then later began to see similar journeys in my patients, my understanding of and appreciation for the connection between our emotions and our health grew. These experiences have changed my life and the lives of my patients forever. It is easy to say "Our emotions affect our health," but to experience it firsthand has given me a totally different perspective than I had before.

There are many people who praise me for healing them, and I always need to correct them. I am not the one who has healed them - their own bodies have. The body has the innate intelligence to heal itself; I am just the facilitator of that healing.

Over the years I have found that there are six major emotions that cause the most problems with my patients' health. They are: ***anger, fear, criticism, self-esteem, resentment,*** and ***forgiveness.*** I realize, of course, that there are many more emotions that can also cause health problems, but these are the most common ones that continue to regularly surface in the patients who come to my office.

These stories of healing would never have come about without the many teachers and mentors who have blessed my life forever. "When the student is ready the teacher will appear" is a Buddhist proverb, but in my case, I have often felt that the teacher appears, and I later discover why I needed that teaching.

Without these great people entering my life, the resources that I have to help the people who come into my office would be limited. Most of the knowledge that I give to others is not mine but that of the teachers I have met throughout my own journey. They have always been gracious in sharing their knowledge with me. This book is my way of returning that favor and sharing what I have learned with others.

My wish is that this book will help you, the reader, to learn more about the effect that emotions can have on your health and your body. I hope that if you experience in your own life something similar to the stories written here you will have a better understanding of how to begin your own healing journey, so that you can find your own balance of body, mind, and spirit.

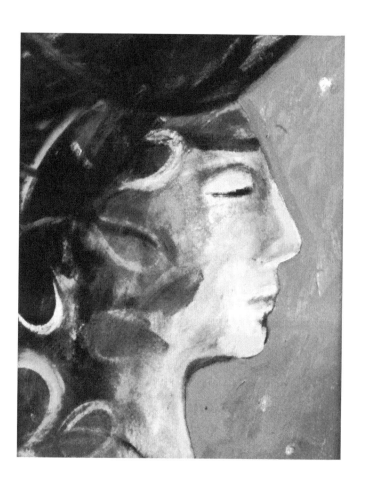

Chapter 1
Anger

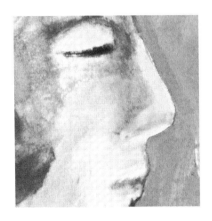

Holding on to anger is like grasping a hot coal with the intent of throwing it at someone else; you are the one who gets burned.

Buddha

The Healer Within

Kristin Malloy entered my office and sat down with a protracted sigh in the wooden chair across from my desk. She looked exhausted. She wore a navy blue suit with gold buttons, a white blouse and low-healed black shoes. She'd obviously just come from work. An identification card still hung around her neck.

While a patient history can give a lot of information, taking the time to talk with a new patient is often a big help in determining a medical issue.

It was 5 p.m. and the 35-year-old was tired from her long, busy day. As we talked, she reached up numerous times to rub the back of her neck or her eyes, as if her head hurt. Kristin looked not only tired but also frustrated. She'd been to so many other healthcare providers and, so far, hadn't found answers to her health problems.

I get a nervous feeling in my stomach when someone comes to see me after going to numerous other medical doctors. It's likely I'm their last resort. They're counting on me to resolve the problem or, at the very least, point them to someone who can. It's a lot of pressure to live up to their expectations, especially if someone I know referred them. I don't want the referring party to be disappointed. To rid myself of this nervous feeling, I take deep breaths and mentally relax.

Earlier in my Chiropractic career, I found myself caring so much about each patient that I was completely drained at the end of the day – emotionally exhausted. I learned to deal with this problem, particularly when it involved referrals, through a woman named Barbara Rose. Barbara is very unassuming. You must spend some time in one-on-one conversations to really get to know her. Barbara was first referred to me by another patient, Linda Smith, who was interested in the metaphysical. One day after treating Linda, she asked me if her friend, Barbara, had come to see me.

"Do you know her?" I asked.

"Oh, she did come to see you. I'm thrilled. I've been telling her that you two really needed to meet!" Linda said.

"Tell me more about her," I asked, surprised at her reaction, because while Linda had referred other patients to me, she had never seemed so excited before.

"She has a great gift for healing," she said, and rattled off a number of different places where Barbara had studied.

Now, when I hear phrases like "a great gift for healing," I tend to take it with a grain of salt, because I often hear similar things about the friends or acquaintances of my patients. What does the phrase "a gift for healing" mean? I've never been sure, but I have learned that often people who are labeled healers are put on a pedestal as if they have something special. The true healer for each of us is ourselves and no one else.

But I was curious, now, about Barbara and her training, so the next time she came to my office I asked her about her experiences. She told me she'd spent ten years in Hawaii learning from the Kahunas, teachers of the ancient Hawaiian healing arts.

"That's interesting," I said to her quietly as I thought to myself, "I still don't buy into this great healing skill Linda told me about."

But each time Barbara returned to my office we talked more about healing and the relationship between the healer and the patient. As our relationship grew, I began to respect her knowledge of people more and more. In fact, I now consider her one of the people who has most influenced the way I practice Chiropractic today.

I joke with Barbara that she reminds me of Mr. Miyagi in *The Karate Kid,* although she tells me she looks nothing like him — she's about 60 years old with white hair. But, of course, it is the relationship between Mr. Miyagi and the Karate Kid that I mean. In the movie, Mr. Miyagi would say something very simple, and at first, Daniel would not understand it. Then he would have an amazing breakthrough as he figured out what Mr. Miyagi really meant. This always happens when Barbara tells me something.

The following is some of the advice she's given me over the years:

•	"Don't care emotionally so much. If you start caring too much it will emotionally exhaust you and block you from really helping people. That's one of the most important things I learned from the Kahunas," she said. I now tell people to look within themselves when looking for healing. "I am just the facilitator who helps you find your own solution to your health problems."

•	"Look for progress, not perfection. If you always look for perfection, you will be let down by the result." This goes for personal growth as well. If you look for perfection, you forget about all the progress you've already made.

•	"Simple things come from God and complex things come from man!" Man is constantly looking for the most complicated solution to a health problem rather than the cause. It is all about ego. Healthcare practitioners often fall into this trap too, and look for something complex that will challenge their skills, rather than something simple.

•	"Always keep your ego in check, because then you will find better solutions," is another of Barbara's mottos. It's often difficult for a doctor to keep it simple, because we worry that patients will think we're doing nothing. It takes a lot of strength on my part to keep away from diagnostic tests and to find a much simpler way of practicing Chiropractic.

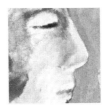

I was reminded of all these things as I looked over Kristin's patient form. I saw nothing unusual in it that would caution me against adjusting her. She suffered from the usual low back problems that many people have. Her biggest complaint was the debilitating migraine headaches which she suffered from every two to four days for the past six months.

"Do you know what brings the headaches on?" I asked.

"I have no idea," she said with a frustrated shake of her head.

"Have you been to see a medical doctor about your headaches? Did they give you a diagnosis?" I asked.

"The medical doctor said it was caused by mini-seizures," she said.

The previous doctor had done the usual tests: blood, urine, x-ray, MRI, and CAT scan, but had not come to a definitive conclusion as to the cause of the headaches. Kristin was frustrated because the medical doctors she'd seen simply gave her pain medications that made her nauseous and sick. It was difficult for her to go to work and, more importantly, live her life normally.

Until the past six months, she'd been a very active person. The headaches and the medications prevented her from participating in many of the physical activities she enjoyed. The only thing that helped her was to sit in a dark room with no noise and an ice pack on her neck. Needless to say, this was awkward, and she was unable to do much of anything with an icepack on her neck all the time. She put up with the excruciating pain day in and day out because nothing seemed to help her. Finally, her sister suggested she visit me because I use a different approach.

"Is there anything else you might have forgotten to tell me that could help me to help you?" I asked.

"Nothing," she replied, and I asked her to move to the other side of the room so I could examine her.

I quickly saw that she was dehydrated and told her to drink three more glasses of water each day. I could also tell that some of her cranial bones were misaligned.

The cranial bones make up the hard covering of the skull. They are joined together by something called sutures, rigid articulations that allow very slight movements of the cranial bones. The very slightest movement out of the normal position can cause devastating affects to a person's health. Many people in the medical community don't believe that the cranial bones can move. They believe these bones are fused and can't possibly move out of place.

Dr. John Upledger, D.O., is the founder of Cranialsacral Therapy. The basis of his approach is that cranial bones can become fixated and not move properly. Once adjusted to move properly, they won't cause health problems. In Kristin's case, the sphenoid bone and the parietal bones were misaligned. This can cause major health problems for a number of reasons.

The sphenoid bone touches every cranial bone in the skull. If it is misaligned it's quite possible that all of the cranial bones in the skull can become misaligned. That is why the sphenoid bone is called the keystone bone. One of the side effects of misalignment of the sphenoid bone and parietal bone is migraine headaches.

I began by adjusting Kristin's lower back and neck region. That seemed to relieve her lower back problems. I adjusted her sphenoid bone, and parietal bone and the migraine headache pain was instantly relieved. I could tell when the headache was gone, because of the look of amazement on Kristin's face. She could hardly believe how quickly the pain had disappeared. Often, it happens so fast that it takes a few moments for the brain to realize what has occurred. Patients are always amazed that such a simple procedure can make such a difference. Of course, this also means that people don't always credit the technique for helping them. In Kristin's case I explained that the adjustment had caused her migraine headache to go away.

"Should I come back?" she asked.

"Yes, in a week we'll see how you're doing."

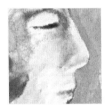

"How are you feeling?" I asked Kristin when she came in the next week.

"The back problems are much better, but the migraine headaches have returned," she said with frustration in her voice. "They're worse than ever this week."

I checked her again and adjusted a few subluxations, or misalignments of the spinal column, that cause nerve interference and prevent the cells, tissues and organs in the body from getting the right messages from the brain.

"How do you feel?" I asked again after the adjustment.

"My migraine is much better now. It's amazing how quickly it goes away when you adjust me, but I'm worried that just like last week, it will come back again," she answered with a look of utter disgust and failure on her face. I could almost hear her saying to herself, "Here we go again. Different doctor, same result."

I had a sudden panic in my heart that I had failed her. I took a breath, refocused and reminded myself of Barbara's words, "Look for progress, not perfection." Kristin's answer and the look on her face told me that I needed to delve deeper to find the real cause of the migraine headaches, and I needed to do it fast if I was going to help her out. The fact that her headaches had returned so quickly also told me that the cause of the problem was not just physical.

I often see this type of thing in my practice. I call it the rebound effect. The physical symptoms go away for a short time, but quickly return, sometimes even worse. The body has many different layers, like an onion. In Kristin's case, I had peeled away the physical layer, and now another layer was showing. The layers can be physical, chemical, or emotional in nature. These three things are the causes of subluxations that are discussed later in this chapter.

Often, in the tougher cases that come to my office, I find there is a different, underlying cause to the problem that has not been addressed by the healthcare practitioners the patient sees before visiting me. Sometimes I get a funny feeling in my stomach, a gut feeling about the cause of the problem. Other times a word, a person or even a name may flash in front of me, and I have a quick idea of the cause of the person's problem. This type of intuition is like a muscle: the more you use it the stronger it becomes.

In Kristin's case ,this intuitive sense was picking up that the cause of the migraines was an emotional trauma that had happened six months before at work, and it had become an ongoing problem.

"You aren't getting along with an older woman in your office, are you?" I asked her.

"Why? How do you know that?" she asked, surprised.

"My intuition is telling me your headaches have an emotional cause. They are coming from your anger at this woman."

"You're right. I do have a problem with someone in my office. Mary is another admin. We have the same pay grade, but she is always acting as if she is my boss. I know she's older than I am and has more experience than I do, but it's not as if I've never done this job before! I'm good at my job, but she gives me no respect. It just makes me so angry, I can hardly say good morning to her anymore without feeling upset."

As she spoke, her voice became more agitated. This was a big stress factor in her life.

"The anger you feel toward your coworker is the cause of these terrible migraine headaches you are experiencing," I said. "Until you release the anger you feel toward Mary, you won't be free from these headaches. I know they are debilitating and you want to get on with your life, but as long as you let her anger you, she will control you."

I described two techniques to help her change the situation. I asked her to work with these techniques for helping her deal with her anger toward Mary, and then come back and see me again.

I was amazed at the difference I saw in Kristin the next time she came to my office. She looked more relaxed, and I could tell just by looking at her that her pain was gone.

"It's really hard," she admitted, "but I'm working on it, because I know it will help my headaches and I want them gone forever. I'm going to keep trying, because I haven't had a headache all week!"

Kristin has been migraine headache-free ever since.

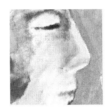

Looking back at this case, I realize that it helped me learn to always listen carefully. My ability to listen and use my intuition began with my friend, Barbara Rose. If I had been unwilling to listen to her ideas because they were new to me, I probably wouldn't have a clear enough mind to manage a case such as Kristin's properly. My intuition might have been blocked or ineffective if I was too busy worrying about the result. Barbara had given me very important information that she'd learned from the Kahunas in Hawaii. I have learned that listening to her and learning from her helps me with many of the problem cases that come to my office.

Anger Releasing Techniques

Spend a few minutes thinking about the person you are angry with, but this time, instead of thinking about the things that anger you or what you dislike about the person, try to come up with three to five things that you admire about her. This will help turn the negative energy that you have for this person into positive energy, and as you focus on these admirable traits, you will forget about the negative things that you dislike.

Of course, the first thing people say to me when I explain this technique is that they can't think of anything they like about the other person. If this is the case, try to start by focusing on very simple things such as she always wears great shoes, or I like her hair. It doesn't matter how simple the things are, just the act of focusing on something constructive will bring that positive energy to you.

The second technique is to try not to take things personally if someone has said something to you that makes you angry. Most likely the person who is saying these mean things is having a problem in their own life.

These techniques may sound simple, because it can be difficult to change your mind about a person and the way in which you deal with situations in which people make you angry. The results, however, are well worth the effort.

What Are Subluxations?

Subluxations are slight dislocations or distortions in the spine and body structure that can cause a serious form of nerve stress as well as physical, mental or emotional malfunction. They are often associated with loss of energy, pain, weakness and disease of all types. Subluxations may be caused by physical, chemical or emotional stress or trauma and can occur in the cranial bones, the vertebral column, sacrum, coccyx, discs, hips, sternum, ribs, femur, shoulders, feet and hands.

As subluxations are corrected, people often experience "retracing" as deep, unhealthy stresses leave the body. This retracing, which is expressing and releasing unhealthy physical and emotional stresses, is an essential aspect of the journey toward health and wellness.

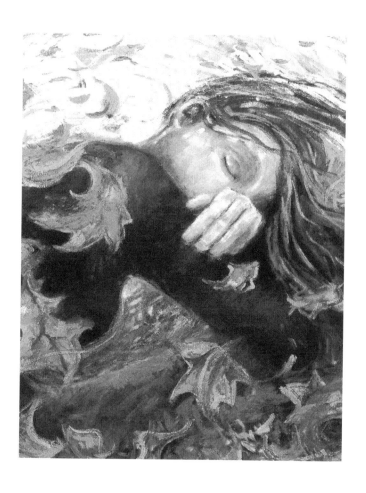

Chapter 2

Fear

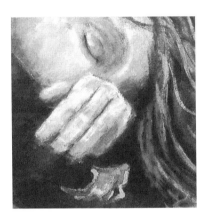

I learned that courage was not the
absence of fear,
but the triumph over it.

Nelson Mandela

Third Eye Blind

"Dr. Kita. How Can I help you?"

My phone had rung during lunch and Kristin, my assistant, wasn't there, so I answered.

"This is Anthony Davis," said a quiet, professional-sounding voice on the other end of the line. I could hear his apprehension, even in just these few words. I've gotten used to it over the years, so it really doesn't bother me anymore. Many people are apprehensive about something they feel is different, and I learned how to deal with being different in my childhood. I was the only Asian in my school.

As an adult that feeling of being different has continued — not because I'm Asian, but because I'm a Chiropractor, and a different one at that. Even some of the other Chiropractors I know find my intuitive work to be "different" enough to make them uncomfortable.

"How can I help you?" I asked, hoping that a calm voice and polite manner would put the man on the other end of the phone at ease. Anthony began to tell me about his daughter, Olivia, who suffered from chronic health problems. He and his wife had taken her to several doctors, but no one could diagnose the cause of her excruciating headaches, dizziness, nausea, and vision problems.

The 16-year-old was often in terrible pain, he told me, and I could hear the distress in his voice. Like any father, he felt helpless and frustrated that he'd been unable to stop his daughter's suffering. They'd seen many top-notch specialists in the area, and I was his last resort. He would bring his daughter to see me, even though he was skeptical that someone who was "just a Chiropractor" could help his child.

Mary Wills, a receptionist at a major insurance company and one of Anthony's coworkers, made the referral. Mary has worked there for many years and knows just about everybody in the company. She is a caring soul and a good listener. While some people might find her garrulous ways nosy, her intentions are always good. She has sent more than 70 people to my office over the years. I'm grateful she believes in the work I do. I've heard from some of her referrals that she doesn't just suggest, she pushes.

"You should go see Dr. Kita before you go to any other doctor, especially if you're thinking about surgery," she says.

"Here we go again," I thought, when I realized that Olivia and her father were a Mary referral. Mary always seems to find me difficult cases. I call them brainteasers. I know her referrals will make me dig deep and use not only all of the things I learned in Chiropractic College, but much more. Besides, it turned out that Olivia was going to be one of my most unusual cases.

Anthony made an appointment for the following week. When I walked into the reception area that afternoon, I saw both Anthony and his daughter wandering around the room, inspecting everything. Their curiosity was palpable.

Too uncomfortable to sit and wait, Anthony stood by the elliptical-shaped coffee table and picked up each of the dozen or so medical pamphlets that were there. He would glance quickly at one, then put it down and move to the next.

I introduced myself to him. He gave me a firm handshake. Then he introduced me to Olivia. She hung her head a little, looking timidly back at me from beneath dark blonde bangs without saying a word. I could feel both pairs of eyes checking me up and down. "What makes him so special? He looks pretty ordinary to me," they both seemed to be silently saying. It made me uncomfortable; I felt like a mannequin in a store window, being gawked at by the passers-by.

They came into my office and perched on the edges of the two teakwood chairs in front of my desk. Anthony handed me Olivia's patient health history form. I looked it over, asking a lot of questions as I read. Invariably, Anthony answered as Olivia sat quietly, looking down at her hands in her lap.

"She's been having terrible headaches almost daily. They start in the front of her forehead and spread all the way around to the back," Anthony said.

I could hear the frustration in his voice as he described how dizzy and nauseous the headaches made her. Her vision was even affected.

"She tells me it feels like she has a net in front of her eyes," he said. "What could be causing this? Olivia's a good student. She wants to go to a good college. She's always made good grades, but these health problems are really starting to affect her work. I'm getting worried that if we don't cure this it's really going to start to affect her GPA," he said anxiously.

The vision problems made it difficult for Olivia to concentrate while the headaches increased her homework time.

"Sometimes it takes her until well after midnight to finish her work. Then she gets to bed late and is tired the next day and that just makes the headaches and the vision problems worse. It's a vicious cycle," Anthony said, shaking his head. I noticed Olivia nodding quietly in agreement.

As I continued to look at her records, I saw that a previous doctor had diagnosed Olivia with Thoracic Outlet Syndrome on her right side, but had been unable to treat it.

Thoracic Outlet Syndrome is compression of the nerves that pass through the neck and the arm, usually causing pain in the arm and the hand. In Olivia's case she felt numbness and tingling in her right hand. I asked her if she had any idea what might have caused this problem with her right hand, and this time she answered for herself.

"I don't know of anything I could have done to cause it," she said in a low voice.

Anthony spoke up quickly.

"Olivia did have two concussions in the last few years," he said. "The first was a playground accident, where she fell off the swings. Neither her mother nor I were with her that day. The second was just last year. She fell during a volleyball game."

Anthony went on saying that Olivia had also been a passenger in three very bad motor vehicle accidents over the past five years, though she hadn't received any specific injuries. After hearing this list of traumas Olivia had experienced, my first thought was that they were the cause of her current problems.

"How many doctors have you already seen for these problems?" I asked.

Five previous doctors: their general practitioner, a pediatrician, an orthopedic specialist, a neurologist, and a special neurologist from the local children's hospital. No wonder they were checking me out so carefully. And no wonder it took Mary such a long time to convince Anthony to bring Olivia in to see a simple Chiropractor. Anthony had taken his daughter to the top specialists in several fields. In his eyes, I couldn't measure up. I had too few letters after my name or diplomas from well-known schools of medicine on my walls.

"Well," I thought to myself, "I think I can help her if they will stick with me, but this is going to be a big learning experience for me." Even as I thought this, I didn't realize just how much I would learn, or how unusual this patient would turn out to be.

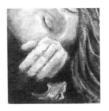

I continued to question Anthony and Olivia about her symptoms for a few more minutes. Then I asked my usual final question.

"Is there anything else you might have forgotten to tell me that would help me in helping Olivia?"

They both said no, so Olivia walked over with me to begin the adjustment. As I began to work, I found she had multiple misaligned cranial bones, which — as in the case of Kristin — can lead to major health problems.

I checked her vision for ocular lock, a neural problem created when the eyes move in certain directions, making the eye muscles weaken and have difficulty following motion. This can make it hard to read. I thought it might be the cause of the teen's vision problems. Ocular lock is often seen in people who have dyslexia.

Our eye muscles are attached to our cranial bones. If these bones have been out of position for a long time, the eye muscles cannot function adequately. Olivia did have ocular lock and I adjusted her to free up the eye muscle movements. Once that was completed, she immediately told me she felt as if she could see better, although her vision was still not where it was before the headaches began.

That was enough for one day, and I asked Anthony to make an appointment for the following week. Both father and daughter seemed perplexed. The adjustments had only taken a few minutes and they were sure that I'd hardly done anything.

"I don't want to wait a week," Anthony said. "I'll bring her back in two days. The faster you work the faster we get her healed."

I explained that although from the outside, it looked as if very little had been done, Olivia's body still needed time to adjust and integrate before I continued. If you go too fast, too deep, you can cause a healing crisis. Anthony made a few more objections, but Olivia finally spoke up.

"Daddy, this is the best I've felt in weeks. Let's just do what the doctor says," she said quietly.

Since his daughter seemed content to go at my pace, Anthony finally agreed and set up the next appointment.

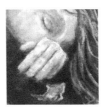

When Olivia and Anthony walked into my office the next week, it was immediately obvious that neither one was happy.

"How are you feeling? Have you seen any changes since your last visit?" I asked.

"Everything was fine for a few days, but then my nausea and dizziness came back. I was so excited because I felt I could be better again when I left here last week, but I think my vision's worse than ever now," she said in her usual quiet voice.

In fact, it was the longest speech I'd ever heard her make. I could hear the discouragement in her voice. I was her last hope, and I could feel that she felt that I was failing. When I was a new Chiropractor, the return of Olivia's symptoms would have alarmed me, even put me in a state of panic. "Oh no, I hope there is no hurt to this girl," I would have thought. But I've learned from experience, and now the return of her symptoms actually gave me a clue to what was really happening with Olivia.

This was another case of Rebound Syndrome. Symptoms disappear after the first visit only to reappear again in a few days. This is often a signal that the underlying cause of the physical symptoms is really emotional. On her first visit, I peeled back one layer of Olivia's problem. Now I could see the second layer, as in the previous chapter with Kristin. I've learned that two layers are usually only a small part of the "onion" that makes up our physical and emotional health. I could tell we were only beginning to see the many layers of Olivia.

During this appointment, I focused my attention on a possible emotional cause, and I allowed my intuition to work. It was telling me that there had been an event the previous June, about six months earlier, and that it involved Anthony's mother. I asked the pair about it.

"That's when my mother passed away," Anthony said quickly, and reached out to touch his daughter's arm. I could see Olivia become tense just at the mention of her grandmother's death.

Traumatic incidents can cause a fear or panic reaction in the body. Watching the reaction of both Olivia and Anthony, I was sure we were beginning to get to the source of Olivia's heath problems.

An emotional or physical trauma can cause a person to put their body in a panic posture. The coccyx or tailbone literally tucks under, just like the tail of a dog when it is scared. The pubic bones move upward to protect the genitals, the sternum or chest moves to protect the lungs and the heart. The larynx moves to a position to prevent the person from speaking. Sometimes the person's body stays in this panic posture, even though the stimulus for the panic has ended. The person holds this position without even realizing it. Now that I understood that this was part of Olivia's problem, I adjusted her for the panic posture. She took a deep breath – so deep that it felt as if all of the air was being sucked out of the room.

"How do you feel now?" I asked.

"Not really any different," she admitted, and again I could hear discouragement in her voice. She wanted so badly for this to work. She was beginning to hope for major improvements at each small adjustment I made.

But rather than discourage me, her answer gave me more information. It was obvious there was still another underlying emotional trauma. I allowed my intuition to work again, and I picked up the next source. A second trauma had occurred sometime around Christmas.

"There's something else," I said to her. "There is something that you saw in the living room of your home. Something really scared you."

Anthony had remained uncharacteristically silent for the last few minutes, but now he stepped in. "What could have scared you in our own living room?" he asked.

Olivia's mouth was hanging open. She was shocked that I seemed to know about the event, even though she'd never spoken about it to anyone.

Olivia stared at us silently for a few moments, then slowly told her story.

"It was Grandma. I saw her. She talked to me. I know it sounds crazy, but I did see her, even though she had been dead for almost six months," she said defensively.

"I'm sure you dreamed it," Anthony said quickly, and glanced at me as if asking me to affirm this innocuous interpretation of the event, rather than the more frightening version his daughter believed.

But I didn't follow his lead. He might have wanted to take the easy way out, but Olivia was obviously certain of what she'd seen. It wasn't going to help to pretend it hadn't happened. "What was it that she said to you?" I asked.

"She said she loved me," Olivia said as she began to cry.

Anthony hugged his daughter, and I could see there were tears in his eyes also. This was a life changing experience for both of them, but I knew there were still more layers to this emotional onion.

"Is this the first time you've seen someone's spirit?" I asked when Olivia had become more calm.

"No," she shook her head.

"She started talking about seeing spirits when she was about five," Anthony said, his arms still around the girl. "We didn't believe her, of course. Well, except maybe my mother. We told her she was just dreaming and as she got older she never said anything else about seeing spirits. We thought it was just a typical case of imagination run wild."

"I didn't see them anymore because I forced myself not too," Olivia spoke up. "I could keep it under control, and I even started believing it had just been nightmares — until Grandma."

"How do you feel now?" I asked Olivia, as she blew her nose and wiped her eyes.

"A lot better," she said.

"Well, come back in two weeks and we'll see how things are progressing," I told them, feeling that we were finally on the right track to getting Olivia healthy again.

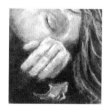

"How are you feeling today?" I asked Olivia as she came into my office on her third visit. Her head was down again, and she seemed almost as shy as the first day I met her, but this time she did answer for herself, rather than letting her father speak for her.

"My vision problems and the terrible headaches are back again, just like before the first visit."

That surprised me. I'd thought that uncovering the emotional portion of her health problems would mean that most of her symptoms would have disappeared at this point. Should I go back to square one, or look for another emotional layer? I knew if the problem still had an emotional cause, it would be buried much more deeply than the ones before. I hoped when I discovered it that it would be the true source of Olivia's health issues. Even as I was thinking this, however, I was also beginning to get the feeling that this time the emotional issue would be something completely new to me.

I had talked with my assistant, Kristin, about Olivia's vision problems a few days earlier.

"Maybe it's a veil," she said.

"What do you mean?" I asked.

"Some people have something that is called a veil, through which they can see spirits," she said.

I'll admit it, before I met Olivia I would have told Kristin to quit the crazy talk. But now I knew better. I have learned to listen to Kristin.

This time, as I checked Olivia's vision problem, I kept the conversation with Kristin in the back of my mind. Olivia said the net she saw was as thick as a heavy rope across her eyes. As I listened, I began to have a gut feeling that Olivia's symptoms involved the chakras, or energy centers, specifically the third eye.

I don't remember where I first learned about chakras, but I'd dealt with this before with other patients. In my experience, if one of the chakras is closed or blocked off, it can cause major health problems. The chakras must always be in balance. I checked Olivia's chakras and, sure enough, the third eye chakra was closed. It told me there was something in her life she did not want to see or visualize.

Usually, when the third eye is closed, it means the person doesn't want to see because a previous emotional trauma that is too painful. I adjusted Olivia to open up the third eye. She immediately began to see better again. This was good news, but I felt cautious about celebrating. What was the correlation between the vision and headache problem and the third eye chakra? I knew we had to figure this out for Olivia's problems to go away once and for all.

I explained the third eye chakra to Anthony and Olivia, and explained that Olivia's had been closed. Both father and daughter looked at me as if I were crazy. I found this amusing. Olivia, after all, was the one who saw spirits.

"The chakras are energy portals that spin to different frequencies or vibrations. They each have their own colors and represent different emotions," I told them. "Eastern philosophy states there are seven chakras and when one is off balance or becomes blocked, it can cause a physical reaction.

Anthony began to nod. He'd become used to my unorthodox way of treating Olivia.

"So far, she's seen more relief after her visits with you than with all these other doctors, so let's go for it," he said.

"I believe Olivia is purposely closing her third eye because she is afraid to see spirits again. Are you scared of the spirits?" I asked.

"Yes," she said, nodding her head emphatically. "Wouldn't you be?"

"I understand, but by trying to forcefully block these forces, your body is just keeping it all inside your head. The consequences are tremendous, because all of this energy from the third eye is held in the skull area, causing these painful headaches and possibly more detrimental health problems in the future.

"You have a gift! Not many people can see what you can. I know it frightens you, but instead, try to realize that this really is a gift. Be happy and embrace, it rather than being afraid. If you continue in this state of fear, the net you see will only get worse," I said.

But Olivia did not want to see spirits. She just wasn't ready. "There has to be some solution," Anthony said.

"Yes, there is another way. Olivia has learned that turning off her third eye keeps her from seeing spirits, but it also has given her headaches and vision problems. She needs to learn not to turn it off forcefully, but in a gentle way," I said.

I hoped Olivia understood what I was telling her, and asked her and her father to come back in one more week.

When she arrived for this fourth visit, I could immediately see a change in her. Her head was up, she met my eye, and she even smiled a bit. She seemed much more relaxed than the first day I saw her. Her headaches were completely gone, and her vision problems had cleared. She had truly learned how to embrace her gift, to gently turn off her visions without causing the physical problems. Olivia and her father left my office knowing that they finally had an answer, and a solution, to her health problems. When she is ready to use her gift, she will also be able to just as gently "turn on" her third eye.

The Seven Chakras
By Kristin Williams

Chakras are energy portals that spin to different frequencies or vibrations. They each have their own colors and represent different emotions. Eastern philosophy states that there are seven major chakras and when one of these goes off balance or becomes blocked, it can then cause a physical reaction.

1.   Root Chakra. The color is red, and the location is at the base of the spine. The root chakra is also known as the mother chakra, and represents family and financial security.

2.   Sacral Chakra. The color is orange, and the location is just below the navel. The sacral chakra is also known as the father chakra or sex chakra. This chakra represents addictions, desires and cravings.

3.   Solar Plexus Chakra. The color is yellow. The location is just below the sternum. The solar plexus chakra represents one's worry, self-esteem, self worth and confidence.

4.   Heart Chakra. The color is green, and the location is in the middle of the chest. The heart chakra represents a person's ability to give and to receive love.

5.   Throat Chakra. The color is light blue, while the location is in the throat. The throat chakra represents expression of speech and creativity.

6.   Third Eye Chakra. The color is indigo blue, and the location is between the brows. The third eye chakra represents a person's ability to see spiritual truth or clairvoyance.

7.   Crown Chakra. The color is violet. The crown chakra floats just above the top of the head. The crown chakra represents one's spirituality. When one transitions to the other side or crosses over from their life, the crown chakra sheds the physical body and the life force energy (or spirit) leaves through it. The crown chakra is also one's ability to communicate with spirits or the divine.

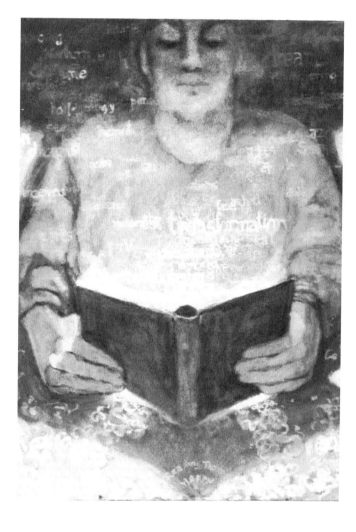

Chapter 3
Criticism

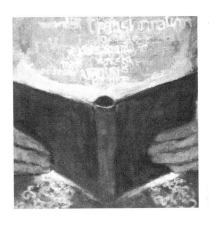

Criticism is an indirect form
of self-boasting.

Emmet Fox

Seeing Red

One day, a patient suggested I check out a New Age metaphysical bookstore in the next town over from my office. She knew I was becoming interested in a variety of metaphysical subjects and thought the books there would help me learn more about intuition and various other subjects.

"Soulutions" is in an old Colonial three story house with a beautiful wooden front porch painted a light blue. Big potted plants decorate both sides of the porch, and baskets hang gracefully from the porch ceiling. When I opened the front door, a set of delicate chimes rang to let the shopkeeper know a visitor had arrived. I was delighted with what I found. The store had many books, CD's, DVD's and other offerings on a wide variety of metaphysical subjects. A store clerk quickly came up to me and asked if I needed help.

"I'm just looking around," I told her.

I wanted some time to explore on my own. One other customer was in the store; a young-looking, athletically-built blonde was browsing through the books in one corner. A book near her caught my interest, and I stopped to leaf through it.

"I could stay here all day and read," I said, looking up from my book.

"I know what you mean," she replied. "I just wish I could read better. It takes me such a long time to read just one book."

"Do you have a problem with reading?"

"I'm dyslexic," she said, with a small smile and a downward glance that told me she was embarrassed to admit her issue.

"Maybe I can help you out. I've had a good bit of success working with dyslexics," I said, and told her a little about my practice.

She seemed very enthusiastic, asking me for a card and promising to call the next day for an appointment. I have to admit that despite her enthusiasm, I was a little bit skeptical that I would ever see her again, and certainly not the next day.

We've all had those chance encounters where we meet someone who promises to call but never does. And in my profession, statistics show that most people won't call right away. It usually takes one or two years for a person to come into a Chiropractor's office after first hearing about him or her.

This time I was wrong. The young woman, her name was Claire Black, went home from the bookstore and called my office. I was quite surprised the next morning when my assistant told me I had a new patient.

"She said she met you at the bookstore and really wanted to start working with you. She seemed so enthusiastic. Since we just had a cancellation I was able to fit her in today," Kristin said.

I was surprised, of course, and happy that she was coming in, but as usual, I felt a little bit of worry and doubt about my own abilities. The quick response to our conversation made it obvious just how much Claire wanted to improve her reading skills. I hoped I could help her.

When I have any doubts, I try to remember some advice from a friend: "Put yourself in as many uncomfortable positions as possible, because that is how you grow, professionally and personally. The more you do this to yourself, the bigger the opportunities that will come to you in the future," he said.

It's a good thing to keep this in mind when I start to worry that a situation, or a patient's problems, are bigger than I can handle. No matter the outcome, both the patient and I will learn from the experience.

Clare arrived about fifteen minutes early, eager to see what I could do for her dyslexia. Well, eager is an understatement, considering I'd just met her the day before.

"You obviously mean business, since I just met you yesterday," I commented as she sat down.

Yes, she was certainly eager. She already had her case history filled out, and I quickly glanced over it. No major health problems existed except for her vision. She had an athletic build, worked out regularly and watched what she ate.

"How long have you had the dyslexia?" I asked.

"Pretty much my whole life. It got worse when I was a teenager, though," she replied.

"Are you having problems looking at words, numbers or both?" I asked.

"When I try to read, the words just seem to get jumbled on the page," she answered with a shrug.

"Hmm," I thought, "This should be a fairly easy case. I don't think she has any other issues." Of course, I should have known better. Thinking like that is always a mistake.

I handed her a book and asked her to read a page so I could see how difficult it was for her.

"It's hard," she answered after looking at the page for several minutes. "The letters seem to be misplaced on the page. It seems like I always have to read the same sentence more than once before I understand what it says."

She put the book down and l began to adjust her. Some of the cranial bones were misaligned, and I adjusted them into place with a light force. I asked her to reread the page in the book I had just given to her.

"The reading flowed so much easier this time. The words didn't feel jumbled! It's like a miracle!" she said excitedly.

Claire was shocked that her dyslexia was removed so quickly after she'd suffered with it for so many years.

"How long will this last? Will it wear off so the words are jumbled again?" she asked worriedly.

"It's hard to tell. Everyone is different. But in my experience it usually goes away forever," I said. "Now that's enough for today's session. I want you to come back for a follow-up visit next week. You don't want me to do too much at one time and mess up what I just did."

Many people confuse the amount of time I spend with them with the amount of healing that takes place. They think if I do not spend a long time with them that they're not getting their money's worth. But when you see a doctor, you are paying for more than just their time – you are paying for their knowledge, experience, and skill. I might spend all day with one person and accomplish nothing, and spend a few minutes with another person and change a life forever.

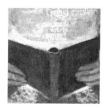

"Have there been any changes since the last time?" I asked when Claire entered my office.

"The dyslexia was only gone for three days," she admitted dispiritedly.

I shook my head, and knew how upset I'd feel in her circumstances. To suddenly be able to read without a struggle, only to have the ability gone a few days later would almost be worse than to never have it all.

"Have you had any trauma to your head in the past week?" I asked.

No, there had been nothing different or unusual to cause her symptoms to reappear.

I began to adjust her. More misalignments had to be addressed before I could look at the dyslexia issue. I knew that once the misalignments were adjusted, I would be able to see if anything else had opened up. My intuition was kicking in. It told me that an emotional issue was causing her vision and reading problems.

"What was your relationship like with your father when you were 16?"

I knew I'd hit a nerve as I saw her body tense. Her shoulders hunched, her head hung down. It was almost as if she took on the posture of a 16-year-old teenager, rather than that of the confident young woman I'd first met in the bookstore.

"He constantly criticized me; nothing was ever good enough. He wanted me to get straight A's all the time and if I got just one B, I was a failure. He was such a perfectionist!" she said with anger in her voice.

In her father's eyes, she was a failure because she was not as good in school as he had been. In his mind, that meant she was not as smart as he was. A very well respected medical doctor in the community, who had graduated from one of the best medical schools in the country, he wanted her to succeed in the same ways that he had. He believed that she had no future if her grades weren't good enough for an Ivy League school.

"He was so critical of me that sometimes I felt I could barely look at him! I was afraid all the time that he would say something, particularly in front of my friends or the family," she confessed.

After we talked I checked her again. Different misalignments that hadn't been there previously now showed up. I adjusted her to take away the emotional charge from her father's past criticisms, and then asked her to read again. She took the book from me, read for few minutes, and then handed it back with a worried look on her face.

"What was wrong?" I asked.

"My vision is corrected again, it is easier to read, but how long it will it last?" she said.

Her fear and anxiety of the criticism she'd received was the source of her reading problem.

"In order for your vision to stay corrected you must change your mindset about criticism of you — from your father or from anybody else," I told her. "When somebody is constantly criticizing you, you have two choices to make. You can take their criticisms as correct, or you can tell yourself how sorry you feel for that person because the problem is with them, not you! People who are always criticizing others often have something going on in their own life that causes them to be negative toward others. Don't take things so personally, because it can give you health problems later down the road. If you take in every negative thing that someone ever says about you, it is just as if you are swallowing poison. I know this is a hard thing for most people to do, but it is important for your health."

Claire listened to everything I had to say, then took a deep breath and nodded.

She came in the next week to tell me that she could see more clearly when she read. "I am making a conscious effort to not take things personally anymore!"

I told her that I was very proud of her for making this difficult change in her life. "Not everyone can do this. This will literally change the way you see things and also how you deal with future criticisms from other people."

More on Cranial Subluxations

Your skull is not a single bone; it is made up of many cranial bones. Eight larger bones protect the brain while 14 smaller bones make up the lower front of the skull. Cranial bones are not fused. They remain separate and distinct throughout life; each bone has its own unique movement. The spaces between the bones are called sutures, and are filled with connective tissues, nerves and blood vessels.

Proper movement of the cranial bones is essential for health. In fact, a wealth of clinical research shows that if your cranial bones are out of position, in other words if they are locked or subluxated, your physical and mental health will suffer.

Subluxations of the cranial bones can cause a multiplicity of health problems, including dyslexia, TMJ pain, migraines, hearing and balance problems, and many others.

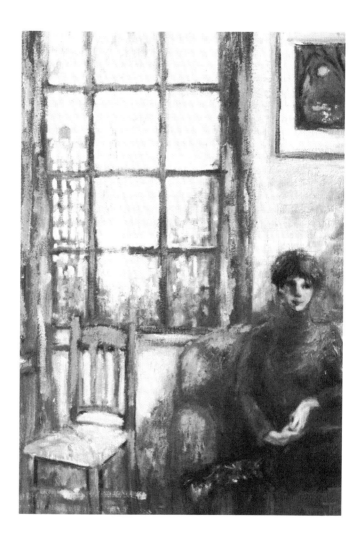

Chapter 4

Resentment

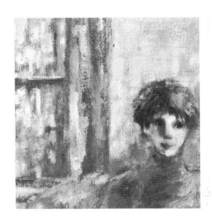

Resentment is like taking poison
and waiting for
the other person to die.

Malachy McCourt

The Resentful Tourist

I was checking the answering machine in my office one morning and found a message from a patient, Anneke, who had been born in Germany. She had an appointment scheduled for that day and was home with her sister, who was in the States visiting for only one month. Could her sister also see me during her appointment time?

I quickly called her back and told her I could fit them both in at one o'clock that day, even though that was during my lunch break. If her sister was willing to take time out from her vacation for a visit to a doctor, I knew she must need help, and I wanted to make sure that I had enough time to take care of them properly.

"Thanks Dr. Kita, we will be over to your office at 1 p.m. today! I'm so glad you can fit my sister in. Brigitte is really having trouble with her shoulder, and I told her I was sure you could help her," she said.

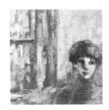

When the sisters arrived that afternoon, Brigitte had a big smile on her face, and told me how eager she was to see me.

"Anneke has said such wonderful things about you. I know you can help me," she said.

It made me a little uncomfortable, because I am just an ordinary Chiropractor. Brigitte wanted her health back. Could I give it to her?

Brigitte was about five-foot-seven-inches tall with blonde hair and a slim, athletic build. I could see the family resemblance between the two sisters, although Anneke was a little taller. They both enjoyed a number of physical activities, particularly hiking, which helped to keep them in shape. After working with Anneke, I went over Brigitte's case history with her. She had a chronic left shoulder problem.

"When did it begin to bother you?" I asked.

"About two years ago," she said.

"Did you have an injury? Was there anything significant you can think of that triggered the problem?" I asked.

"There is nothing I can think of," she replied. "It just seemed like I woke up one day and it hurt. It never gets any better no matter what I do."

Brigitte had seen a number of doctors, but none had any answers for her, either about the cause of the problem or how to relieve the pain that she was feeling. She had been diagnosed with a "frozen shoulder," but given no solutions. She'd been in pain for two years, and by the time she visited her sister, she was beginning to feel pretty desperate, wondering if she would have to live with pain for the rest of her life.

"Anneke wanted so much for me to come to see you," she said. "I think I have nothing to lose at this point, so go ahead and try."

I finished asking questions and told her it was time for me to examine her before starting to adjust her. I checked the range of motion in both shoulders. She could barely lift her left arm an inch or two without pain. The lack of movement was so severe, it crossed my mind that she might be faking it. I thought it was impossible for someone to have such a limited range of motion. I didn't want to confront her about her faking the shoulder problem though, until I learned more. People who are just looking for attention will often exaggerate their symptoms to get attention from their friends and family. A health problem serves as something for them to always talk about, and make them the center of attention.

But to learn if a person is really in pain or is faking, I initially must take their complaint seriously. It is unfair to accuse someone of pretending to be hurt without first doing everything I can to help them. I adjusted her and she told me she felt better throughout her body, except for her shoulder. There was only slight improvement there; her range of motion was still far from normal.

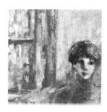

Since Brigitte's time in the States was limited, I set an appointment for her to return only a few days later. No signs of significant improvement appeared in her shoulder over the few days since I had previously seen her, and as I listened to her, my intuition began to tell me that this problem was more than physical.

"A woman has been taking advantage of you, right?" I asked.

Anneke, who had come to the appointment with her sister, nodded even as

Brigitte shrugged her shoulders as if to say, "It's no big deal."

I knew I'd hit on something though, and with a little prodding from Anneke, Brigitte began to tell me her story.

"I'm a tour guide in Germany, you see. We take bus tours throughout the country, and as the guide I try to do much more than just tell my people the history of what they are seeing. I go out of my way to find stories about the places, to make them come alive for the people. I want them to love Germany the way I do," she said with passion. "I find the best cafes to recommend for them to have lunch and the little shops where they will find more than just the usual souvenirs.

"There are always two buses on the tour, mine and my boss's. And my bus is always full, while hers is half empty. Even if we start out with the same number of people on each bus, by the end of the trip, as many as possible have moved over to my bus.

"I don't mind, in one way. I'm proud of being good at what I do, and proud of the fact that the tourists want to be in my bus, but what it means is I'm the one who is always doing most of the work, but I'm the one who is making less money. My boss sets my salary, and she hasn't given me a raise in two years. I'm the person who is making the most money for the company, but I'm getting paid the least!"

As she told me her story, she spoke faster and more passionately with each sentence.

"Yes, we've found something here," I thought. In fact, Brigitte had first asked for a raise and been denied just a few weeks before her shoulder pain began. I now knew I needed to adjust Brigitte to rid her of the emotion of resentment which was the root cause of her shoulder pain.

Resentment is rather like playing an old record that has a scratch in it. You put the record on the turntable, place the needle down and you begin to listen to the music, but then you get to the scratch and the needle skips. It just keeps playing the same phrase of the song over and over again. When we feel resentment against a person it's just like playing that old record. We go along fine throughout the day, but as soon as we think about the person we resent, we get stuck. To move forward with our song, we have to pick the needle up and move it beyond the scratch. We have to move beyond the resentment.

"It's good that you could explain this to me," I told Brigitte. "Now I know that I need to find out what part of your body is blocking your healing energy. When we unblock the energy, it is like picking up the turntable needle and moving beyond the scratch in the record. You'll be able to move beyond your resentment."

I could certainly identify with Brigitte's problem, as I'd recently had a similar experience. Someone had been using me to bring many clients to his own business while giving me no help in my own. It seemed that the more I gave, the more this man took, without ever thanking me or acknowledging in any way the help I was giving to him.

I was sick and tired of it. Sometimes it seems as if we must reach a breaking point before we take responsibility for a problem in our lives. I knew I'd gotten myself into this problem, and I had to take responsibility and get out of it. I told him, "No more."

The same was true for Brigitte. I adjusted her to get rid of the emotion of resentment she was feeling, and I was not surprised to find that the block was in her right hip. There is a theory that our subconscious lies in our hips. Why? I don't know, I just know that often when emotion is blocked, this is where the adjustment must be made. As I finish an adjustment, I usually see the patient take a deep breath as the anxiety is released.

While Brigitte felt better the instant I made the adjustment, I told her to return for a few more appointments while she was in the United States. This way I could reinforce the healing process. I also knew that unless she dealt with the problem with her boss, her shoulder pain would return.

"You have to deal with this," I said. "You have to talk to your boss about your feelings, and if nothing comes of the conversation, I suggest you look for another job. It is your responsibility to get yourself out of the situation that is affecting your health.

Brigitte looked at me attentively as I spoke. I knew that she realized that she either had to change how she saw her boss or change her place of employment. It would be a difficult decision either way, but she knew that a change needed to take place, and soon, because her health came first.

Living in
a Stress-Filled Body

Over time, continuous, unresolved nervous tension can cause a buildup of stress hormones in our bodies, making us aggressive, anxious, over-reactive, irritable and hyper-vigilant.

Eventually, a person who is in this state has less energy and a weakened immune system which can often lead to various stress-related disorders such as heart disease, headache, sexual dysfunction, insomnia, high blood pressure, chronic fatigue, depression, rheumatoid arthritis, lupus, allergies, premature aging and more.

Turning to drugs and surgery to suppress symptoms of stress generally means that the body and the mind continue to deteriorate, even though superficially, we feel fine.

Fortunately, an increasing number of people are turning toward the natural, drug-free, non-surgical "alternative" approaches that seek to reduce stress levels and strengthen our ability to handle stress. Yoga, meditation, exercise, nutrition, psychotherapy, herbs, homeopathy, acupuncture, massage, shiatsu, and Chiropractic are all ways in which we can deal with stress.

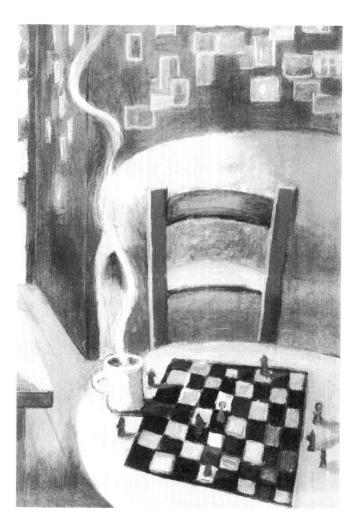

Chapter 5

Forgiveness

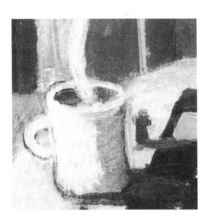

Forgiveness is not always easy. At times, it feels more painful than the wound we suffered, to forgive the one that inflicted it.

Marianne Williamson

Gone, But Not Forgotten

It was a hot summer day, and Mary Munders, a longtime client of mine, came in with a man that I have never seen before. He looked like an aged sailor from one of those old movies that we watched in our childhood days. By just looking at him, I could tell he'd lived a rough life. His skin was wrinkled like leather, probably from working hard outdoors in all sorts of weather. He didn't look particularly healthy – skinny rather than thin or wiry, and I thought he was probably in his 70s.

In contrast, Mary is a young-looking 50. She's petite and fit. She works out a lot because, at only five-foot-two, she knows that even a small amount of weight gain will show. She introduced her companion as her brother-in-law, Paul. She hoped I could help him with a variety of health problems, but especially prostate cancer. I asked him to fill out our new patient forms while I adjusted Mary.

When it was time for him to come into the inner office and talk with me, I could tell he was reluctant. "What the hell is this Chiropractor going to do for me?" was written all over his face. But I could also see that not only was he fond of Mary, he respected her opinions. Since she asked him to come with her, he was willing to give me a try.

"Besides," he told me, "No one else has been able to help me."

As I asked him about his past health history, I could see his eyes wandering around the room. He checked out the degrees, certificates and awards that are on the walls of my office. He wanted to make sure I knew what I was doing before he would trust me to help him. He told me he'd been diagnosed with prostate cancer about a year before. He'd undergone chemotherapy but had seen no improvement. The cancer was still there.

He also mentioned he was a former heroin addict, but had been clean for several years. That explained a number of things, particularly why he looked much older than his age of 50. Often, heroin is cut with sugar before it is injected into the body, and this is one of the reasons it causes premature aging. He'd also had a hard time holding down a job because of his drug addiction. He hadn't taken care of his body and health for many years.

Even though Paul was no longer an addict, he still didn't have a full time job. He was only able to come to see me because Mary had driven him. He didn't have transportation, and he had very little money.

"I've got more important things to worry about than cancer," he told me, "like finding a job. And I can't work because of my back problems."

As I looked over his health history, aside from the prostate cancer, he was in surprisingly good health for a man who had spent much of his life abusing or ignoring his body. I'm not saying that prostate cancer isn't serious of course, just that considering everything, Paul had said about his life, I would have expected him to have had a major health crisis much sooner.

As I started to adjust him I found that his pelvic area was misaligned. The low back pain disappeared quickly as I made the adjustment. Paul was pleasantly surprised. Most people are, so to me, this is not a big deal. Patients tend to visit Chiropractors for the wrong reason: their pain. Chiropractic is about being adjusted so your body will function at its optimum. I was certainly happy to give him some immediate relief from his back pain, but I also wanted to move on to something bigger – the cause of his cancer.

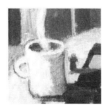

My intuition was telling me something. I have learned over the years that patients often do not want to hear what I have to say. And just as often, my intuition about the receptivity of the patient is accurate. When I first began my practice, I would sometimes just blurt out what I was coming up with without regard for the mental state of the patient. That is usually a big mistake.

In the few times this happened, I had to take a few steps back before I could move forward again with the patient. I've learned to make sure the person is ready to hear what I say and accept it in a positive manner. I am only saying these things to help the person out, and I try to make sure that they understand this before I speak. What came to me about Paul were the emotional problems caused by his father's abuse and abandonment at age 16.

"You're right," he said, when I mentioned it. "But what does that have to do with my cancer?"

I adjusted his right ilium to return the energy from this emotional trauma back into motion.

"You need to forgive your father. If not, you will still feel this emotional upset," I said. "Is he still alive?"

"No, he's not. How can I forgive him if he isn't around anymore?"

It turned out that Paul's father was buried nearby.

"When you leave here, go to his grave and tell him you forgive him for what he did to you," I suggested.

"I don't think I can ever forgive him. It's his fault, all of it. I wouldn't have gotten on drugs if it weren't for him and the way he treated me as a kid. I can't forgive, and I can't forget. He ruined my life," he said.

But forgiveness isn't something you do for the person who has hurt you. Forgiveness is something you do for yourself. Forgiveness doesn't mean you forget the past. That's something that many people don't understand. Forgiving doesn't mean that you pretend that something never happened, or that you should put yourself in a position to be abused or taken advantage of again.

"Forgive your father for yourself – to help yourself heal and get over the emotional trauma," I told Paul. "And remember, I said forgive. Not forget. You should always forgive, but you should never forget. If you forgot about the pain, you would lose the lessons you learned from it. Your father abused you. You learned never to let anyone else abuse you.

That's a good lesson, even if it was learned in a painful way."

There is a saying, "Time heals all wounds." I believe this is totally false. Time doesn't always heal a wound. Sometimes it just prolongs the hurt, and that pain then becomes a snowball, rolling down the hill getting larger and larger until it becomes a much bigger problem.

"Now is the time to get rid of the old hurt," I told Paul. "This is the cause of your cancer. This is the time to free yourself from this bondage." Forgiveness, I told him, is like throwing up. "You don't want to swallow this emotional vomit again do you?"

He gave me a look of disgust at that analogy, but he heard me. He didn't want to swallow that pain again. I also told him that if he didn't take care of an emotional trauma, it would go much deeper into the body. Next time it tries to come out, it will not be a pretty sight. I suggested he go to his father's grave and pretend to talk to him as if he were alive.

"Have a conversation with him and forgive him for what he did in the past, then try writing a letter to him explaining the impact his behavior has had on your life. Explain it to him without blaming him," I said.

In letters of forgiveness it is best to use "I" statements such as "I feel____," or "I don't understand____." After you're satisfied with what you have written, burn it. This is a symbolic way of letting old angers go up in smoke.

"Paul," I said, "now is the time to take responsibility for the past so you can look toward the future."

I'd given Paul a lot to think about, and I knew I'd done and said enough for one visit. I asked him to return in two weeks.

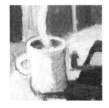

When Paul came in for his next appointment, he looked quite different than he had the first day. His facial expression, his whole demeanor, was relaxed rather than closed in and suspicious.

"Did you do as I suggested? Did you work at forgiving your father?" I asked.

"Yeah, I did. I went out to the cemetery and had a long talk with him. I didn't really think it would help, but when I was done, it felt like someone had lifted a weight right off my shoulders." he said.

"This isn't automatically going to cure your cancer, you know, but it is a great start. It can often take days, weeks, or months before you feel the full effect from the release of the emotional toxins you were storing in your body, but it will always come to pass." I said.

When you deal with toxic emotions, it takes time for the body to cleanse the chemical toxins you have released into your body. Watch your diet, and make sure you drink plenty of water to flush these toxins out.

Three months later, Paul came back to see me. He'd received his most recent test results, and they showed he was cancer-free. It was truly a miracle. I learned something from Paul's experience, myself. It is best to forgive, not only others, but also yourself. Otherwise it can manifest itself into a physical problem.

Without Forgiveness You Become What You Have Not Forgiven

When someone comes to my office with cancer, 100 percent of the time I find they need to forgive someone or they need to forgive themselves.

When you think about it, this is logical. What are cancer cells? The word cancer means "out of control growth." In other words, cancer cells are just normal cells that have begun to grow uncontrollably. A cancer is similar to a break in a personal relationship. In a broken relationship you can no longer communicate with the other person. To move forward, you must forgive that person and make the relationship whole again. Lack of forgiveness fragments the body. Being in a state of unforgiveness can also cause high blood pressure, coronary artery disease, and a decreased immune system, making you vulnerable to many other illnesses.

There are many different people who have taught me things about forgiveness. Harboring feelings of blame or ill will against another person keeps you from moving on with your own life. Forgive the past to move forward. Forgiveness will heal all wounds. Forgiveness is a part of all religions. Many people call this "The Law of the Universe," or to use a more common phrase, "what comes around, goes around."

If someone has hurt you in any way, you have choices. The first is to harbor feelings of ill will toward the person and to refuse to forgive them. In the short term, you may feel more powerful by holding onto the anger and hurt, but there is a problem with this choice. It turns your body and your spirit into a garbage dump for the anger and resentment that you feel.

If forgiveness feels so good, why do so many people carry the burden of hurt and resentment throughout their lives? Because people confuse forgiveness with being weak and wimpy, but they are wrong. It takes focused courage to do! Forgiving will actually give you a greater sense of power. When you forgive, you reclaim your power and control over what you want to happen in your life from now on. To forgive someone for something they have done doesn't mean that their actions were right. Forgive the person, not the deed. You need to constantly forgive in order to remove the layers and finally get to the seed of the problem. If you still feel emotionally charged or attached to your anger, more forgiveness needs to happen. Forgiveness is a continual thing that always needs to be experienced.

Finally, at the end of each day, say to yourself: "If I have offended anyone in thoughts, words or deeds, please forgive me. If anyone has offended me in thoughts, words, or deeds, please forgive them."

God is not judgmental; forgive the other person and forgive yourself. The people you forgive may never know that you were hurt by them, and they may never know that you forgave them. It is often difficult to forgive someone who has hurt us. In the short term it can feel better to harbor our anger. But the things that we don't want to do are often the things that we must do – for our body, our mind and our spiritual health.

You should forgive; otherwise this lack of forgiveness can manifest itself into a physical problem. It really doesn't matter if someone deserves forgiveness. Instead, understand that *you* deserve to be free from the bondage that not forgiving someone can create.

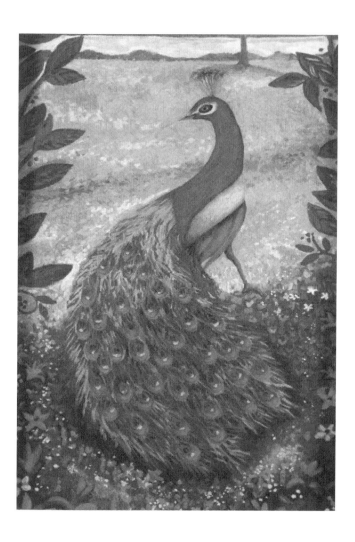

Chapter 6
Self-Esteem

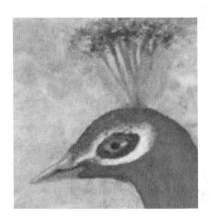

Self- esteem is the greatest sickness
known to man or woman
because it's conditional.

Albert Ellis

Groundhog Day

I had just finished adjusting Lori Ward, and she was telling me how happy she was with the result. Lori had been coming in for the past month. When she first came under my care, she didn't think too highly of my skills. She felt that I was doing nothing for her. Then, after a few weeks, it seemed to her as if all of a sudden the physical problems she was having went away, and she became very happy.

"Why did it take a whole month for me to feel this change?" she asked me.

"Sometimes, there are other issues that need to be addressed before the major issues can be resolved," I said. "It's like a puzzle where you must put all the smaller pieces into place before you can see the bigger picture at the end."

I'd gained some trust with Lori, and she was confident in what I could do to help people. In fact, she was so confident that she decided to bring her daughter, Kim, to see me.

"What kind of results do you have with shoulder problems?" she asked. "My daughter has a frozen shoulder."

"Frozen shoulder is something I've had good results with. But of course, no one can ever give a 100 percent guarantee that they can resolve a problem – particularly before they have seen the patient. And you have to remember, I'm not the one who heals the body. The body knows how to heal itself. I adjust the body to let it function at its optimum. Please don't confuse me as the one who is doing the healing," I said.

"The body's innate intelligence heals the body. When people say to me, 'Dr. Kita, you're such a great healer,' I try and explain this to them. I am just a facilitator that helps the body heal itself." Lori made an appointment for Kim for the following week.

When Kim came for her appointment, I introduced myself to her, and I was impressed by how tall and good-looking she was. She was beautifully dressed, and carried herself in a way that I thought exuded self-confidence. "She must have it all together in her life," I thought to myself.

She sat down at my desk, and we went through the preliminary questions and answers about her past health history. Her main complaint was that she had a chronic right shoulder problem. It had bothered her for the past five years. She felt as if she had seen every health care practitioner in the state for this problem and still had absolutely no relief. I was her last resort.

"I've been diagnosed with frozen shoulder," she said. "And the doctors say the only way to correct it is with surgery."

She had resigned herself to this even though she desperately did not want to have surgery unless there was no other way to fix the problem.

I listened to her story, and then said, "Once you change the structure of a body part you change the function. Surgery changes the structure of the body, and it is hard to reverse a surgery once it is done."

I started adjusting her and found that there were misalignments behind the right shoulder blade. I adjusted the middle back area, and that seemed to release the right shoulder. It caught me off guard when the problem cleared up so quickly. Kim was, of course, thrilled to have her symptoms improve so quickly, but I had a suspicion that this case wouldn't be so easy. I didn't think we had yet uncovered the main cause of the problem, but I couldn't adjust anything else just then.

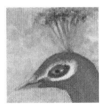

Kim came back the next week. As I'd suspected, her right shoulder problem had returned. I immediately realized the underlying cause of her frozen shoulder was an emotional trauma from her past. Unless she could release it, she would continue to have this problem.

I started adjusting her again, and again her right shoulder began to move properly. This time I wanted her to hold the adjustment without the pain and discomfort returning. As I adjusted her, I felt a sense of loss coming from her body. I had the feeling of the break up of a relationship with a boyfriend, about five years before. I also picked up that he had been the one to break off the relationship. The major emotional trauma that was coming up during the adjustment was that this had been a severe blow to her self-esteem.

I told her what I was picking up.

"How do you know that?" she asked. "Did my mother say something to you?"

"No, she never mentioned it."

As we discussed the situation, she found it difficult to admit that her underlying feeling about the break-up had been a loss of self-esteem.

I always try to put myself in the place of the person I'm talking with. It gives me a much better perspective when dealing with difficult personal issues. I try to make the other person feel more comfortable about him or herself when discussing something so personal and that has made them feel embarrassed and vulnerable.

One of the best examples to use to take the charge off discussing a self-esteem issue is public speaking. The number one thing that most people fear is speaking in public. It is not the fear of talking, because everyone can speak. Instead, the real fear is that we will embarrass ourselves by saying something wrong, or by making a fool of ourselves in front of a lot of people. If everybody had high self-esteem, no one would be embarrassed about speaking in public. This example seems to calm everyone down. They can relate to the public speaking scenario, and it makes them feel a little less vulnerable to realize that at some time in their lives, everyone feels this same lack of confidence in themselves.

In Kim's case, I adjusted her right scapula to remove the energy block from the emotional problem. As I did, something else came to me about Kim and another, earlier emotional trauma. It turned out that several years before that break up, she had experienced another break up.

"That wasn't the first time you had a relationship that ended badly, was it?" I asked.

"No, it wasn't. It's happened to me before," she said.

As we talked, I remembered something my friend, Barbara Rose, had mentioned to me recently. The last time I visited with her, she told me about Kharmic Pattern.

Many people believe kharma to be the law of cause and effect. They see it as meaning that whatever you give, you will receive in return. But a Kharmic Pattern is a little different. In this context, it means the unresolved emotional issues that a person must overcome.

Barbara told me an emotional problem can return over and over again, because the person did not learn the lesson from the first incident. The emotional upset just keeps repeating itself until the person learns from the problem and lets it go. As I explained this to Kim, she mentioned that, yes, there had been a third break-up of a personal relationship in her life. In fact, she'd had three break-ups at approximately five-year intervals throughout her life.

"This is a Kharmic Pattern," I told her. "You need to release this trauma to move forward in your life, or it will continue to happen over and over again."

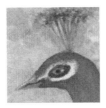

This emotional pattern had already caused her a chronic shoulder problem. If she didn't release it, I said, it could cause an even more serious disease later in life. I adjusted her to break up the kharmic pattern and help her to keep it from happening again.

But adjusting her could only go part of the way in keeping Kim from experiencing similar problems in the future. She also needed to work on building up her self-esteem to rid herself of the past emotional traumas. I asked her to do some self-esteem exercises.

After three months of work, her shoulder pain permanently disappeared and

Kim had become a different, and much more confident, person. She even began a relationship with a new boyfriend, and this time, she confided in me, she could already see a difference in the way she interacted with him because of her newfound confidence in herself.

Mirror Work

I generally ask patients who come to my office for self-esteem issues to participate in something that I call mirror work.

The person doing this exercise should stand and look into a mirror, looking straight into their own eyes. As they do this they should say this simple sentence out loud to themselves three times:

"(*Your Name*), I truly love and accept myself as I presently am."

I ask the person to say this sentence three times at the beginning of each day, and again, three times right before they go to bed, so that they can "sleep on it."

When doing Mirror Work the important part of this exercise is to make sure that you look straight into your own eyes. Don't look to the side of the mirror; look at yourself. This exercise will not work over night. It takes time for a person to build up self-esteem, but it is well worth it.

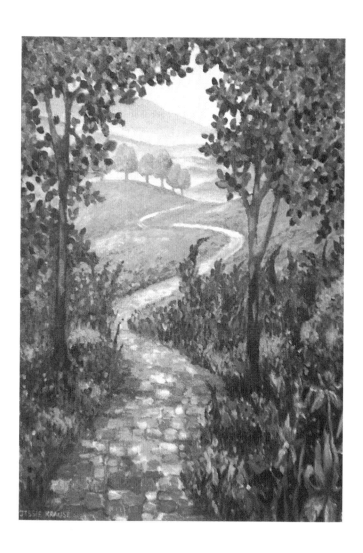

Conclusion

Heal the present
for a better future.

I hope that reading this book has given you some insight into how powerful emotions can be, and just how much effect they can have on your body, mind and spirit. The one common thread that ties each of these stories I have told here is that the people who came to me for assistance had allowed another person or outside force to take control of their lives.

I hope that reading these stories will help you to take a very candid look at your own life and to assess where you are presently in your healing journey. Are you happy with yourself physically, mentally, and spiritually? Remember that you are where you are, and who you are, today because of past decisions or past actions that you have made in your life. There is no better time to change then now! The only things that each of us can control are our own feelings and emotions. We cannot change what other people do; what we can change is how we react to people and to situations.

Don't let anyone else take control of your life! In my office, I see many people who have not taken responsibility for their own health and wellness. They believe that an unknown, outside force – a new doctor, the latest medication, a different die – will somehow, suddenly, make them well, and they passively wait for that day to come. Unfortunately it just doesn't work that way. You, yourself, must take full responsibility for every action and decision you make. Once you do you will see how freeing it will be to your own well-being. Not only will this new attitude help you to heal yourself, you will also become a much more successful person in any other endeavor you take on in the rest of your life.

Everybody has a healing journey, no matter how big or small it may be. When I began this book I did not realize that not only was it about the journeys of my patients, it became a part of my own healing journey and what I needed to learn myself, as well. But that does not mean that *Healing Journeys: Stories of Mind, Body & Spirit* is about me; it is about the people who have come into my office over the years to teach me lessons that I needed to learn, so I could grow and pass them onto others. Every one of these stories is really a mirror of what I needed to learn about myself. I mentioned this to one of my patients recently, and she remarked that what I was describing is called "counter-transference," a word first used by Sigmund Freud. This term explains the phenomenon where the person who is being observed helps the observer become healed at the same time as the person who is being treated.

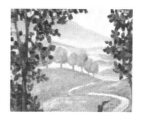

Once we remove our egos, and look deep inside ourselves we see how powerful we are meant to be. If I had not become more receptive to learning new things, the lessons that I learned would never have come about, and this book would never have been written. B.J. Palmer , a pioneer of Chiropractic said, "As ego expands, mind contracts." I could not have accepted the people who have come into my life, or the lessons that they have taught me over the years if I had allowed my ego to get in the way. Every morning I say a simple prayer: "Please God, do not let my ego get in the way of what You are about to give me this day."

I hope that you have read this book with an open mind, and learn from some of the lessons that my patients learned in the stories that I tell here. If you do, you will begin to "grow though life," instead of just "going through life."

The tools that are described at the end of each chapter in this book are so simple that most people will not believe that they actually work. But they do! I have used them in my own personal life, and I have helped countless others to use them, also. So many people read books filled with sound advice, but never use it in their own lives. Someone once told me that is called "poor shelf esteem."

When you read this book, make a conscious effort not to just try these tactics once or twice, but to go out and actually use them every day. In *Healing Journeys: Stories of Body, Mind & Spirit*, some of the tools that I discuss take time. Don't be discouraged if you don't see a change right away. Look for progression, not perfection. Changing the way we deal with the people and the situations in our lives is just like starting to exercise to get into better physical shape. You will not see a difference after just one workout, but over a period of time, if you continue to exercise, you will see a positive difference in yourself.

About the Author

Dr. Kevin Kita D.C., graduated from Sherman Chiropractic College in 1998, and has been in private practice for the past 15 years.

He has served as the Chiropractor for the professional minor league men's basketball team, the Trenton Shooting Stars. He is also an international speaker on the benefits of regular Chiropractic care and a teacher of Chiropractic. In addition to his Chiropractic practice and his speaking duties, he served for several years as the publisher for an internationally recognized Chiropractic newsletter.

Dr. Kita works in Morrisville, Pennsylvania, and is involved in a number of non-profit organizations.

More information on Dr. Kita, his Chiropractic practice and his book, *Healing Journeys: Stories of Mind, Body & Spirit*, can be found at www.Dr.KevinKita.com.

About the Artist

Jessie Krause studied art at Smith College and New York University, then worked as a scenic designer for theater and film while continuing to develop as a painter. While living on Manhattan's historic Gramercy Park, she adopted the square and surrounding sidewalks as her own personal studio, capturing it in hundreds of paintings and drawings that became the basis for her nationally-sold line of greeting cards.

Her work can be found in the collections of the National Arts Club, The Players Club, and New York Life Insurance, as well as a number of celebrities.

Jessie now has a gallery, Netherfield, in New Hope, PA. Her work can also be found on her website at www.jessiekrause.com

35113834R00070

Made in the USA
Charleston, SC
27 October 2014